HEALTHY EATING GUIDE

Eat Healthy For People Who Want To Lose Weight And Improve Their Wellbeing

Eugene G. Davis

Table of Contents

CHAPTER1

What are natural foods

Regular food sources have become progressively famous lately as individuals become more wellbeing cognizant and mindful of the significance of good nourishment. Foods that do not contain artificial ingredients like preservatives, additives, or flavors are considered natural foods. They are also minimally processed. All things considered, they are produced using entire, regular fixings, like organic products, vegetables, entire grains, and lean proteins, the fact that natural foods are typically grown sustainably or organically is another important characteristic. This implies that they are liberated from pesticides, herbicides, and other hurtful synthetic compounds that can hurt both the climate and our wellbeing. Natural cultivating likewise advances biodiversity and supports neighborhood networks, making it an additional feasible and moral decision. In conclusion, natural foods are those that have undergone minimal processing, do not contain any artificial additives, or contain only a small number of synthetic ingredients. They are commonly connected with entire, natural food varieties like organic products, vegetables, entire grains, nuts, and seeds. Regular food sources are additionally normally natural or reasonably developed, advancing biodiversity and supporting neighborhood networks. We can support a food system that is more ethical and sustainable while also improving our health and well-being by choosing natural foods.

In recent years, natural foods have gained popularity, and many people are looking for them to improve their overall health and well-being. Normal food varieties are those that are negligibly handled, and are liberated from counterfeit fixings, additives, and added substances. These foods are frequently organic, which indicates that they were grown without the use of pesticides or chemical fertilizers. Natural foods have become such a popular choice for many people due to their numerous advantages.

Start by including fresh vegetables and fruits in your meals. Vitamins, minerals, and fiber, all of which are necessary for good health, are abundant in these foods. Fruit salad as a snack or vegetables in your omelet or sandwich are two ways to incorporate them into your diet. Natural fruits and vegetables can also be used to make juices and smoothies.

Besides, pick entire grains like earthy colored rice, quinoa, and entire wheat bread rather than refined grains like white rice and white bread. Entire grains are wealthy in fiber and different supplements that are gainful to your wellbeing. You can trade your standard pasta for entire wheat pasta, utilize earthy colored rice rather than white rice, and pick entire wheat bread rather than white bread.

Select lean proteins like fish, chicken, beans, and lentils with care. These proteins are high in nutrients like iron and zinc while being low in fat. You can include fish at least twice a week, eat grilled chicken for dinner, and add beans and lentils to soups and stews.

Natural food consumption is an easy and efficient way to improve your health. You can give your body the essential nutrients it needs to work properly by eating fresh fruits and vegetables, whole grains, and lean proteins. Rolling out these improvements to your eating regimen can assist you with keeping a solid weight, diminish your gamble of persistent illnesses, and lift your energy levels..

CHAPTER2

The advantages of natural foods

Natural foods have become such a popular choice for many people due to their numerous advantages.

One of the main advantages of natural foods over processed ones is that they are much healthier. Regular food varieties are plentiful in nutrients, minerals, and different supplements that are fundamental for good wellbeing. They are also low in fat and calories, making them a great option for people who want to lose weight or keep their weight in a healthy range. Additionally, because they do not require costly packaging or advertising campaigns, natural foods frequently come at a lower cost than processed foods. Natural foods have the added benefit of being better for the environment. Crop rotation and natural pest control are two examples of environmentally friendly, sustainable farming practices that are frequently used to produce natural foods. Additionally, they are frequently sourced locally, which reduces the environmental impact of transportation. Additionally, biodegradable packaging is frequently used to package natural foods, reducing waste and pollution. In conclusion, people who want to improve their nutrition and lessen their impact on the environment can choose natural foods because they are healthy, reasonably priced, and friendly to the environment. We can support local farmers, reduce our carbon footprint, and improve our health and well-being by choosing natural foods. Natural foods are those that have been minimally processed or refined, do not contain any artificial additives, and do not contain any synthetic ingredients at all. There is no regulated definition of the term "natural," and numerous interpretations of what constitutes a natural food exist. However, whole, unprocessed foods like fruits, vegetables, whole grains, nuts, and seeds are typically associated with natural foods. There are a number of factors to consider when defining natural foods. First and foremost, normal food varieties are ordinarily liberated from counterfeit flavors, additives, and tones. Additionally, they lack synthetic ingredients like hydrogenated oils, genetically modified organisms (GMOs), and high fructose corn syrup. Natural foods, on the other hand, are made of whole, minimally processed ingredients that are as natural as possible.

One of the primary advantages of eating regular food sources is that they are a lot more grounded than handled food varieties. Normal food sources are in many cases a lot of lower in calories, fat, and sugar than their handled partners. As a result, they are an excellent option for people who want to maintain a healthy diet or lose weight. Additionally, the vitamins and minerals that are necessary for good health are typically much more abundant in natural foods.

Consuming natural foods has the added benefit of being better for the environment. Natural foods are typically grown in a way that is better for the environment thanks to sustainable farming practices. This is due to the fact that natural farming practices do not rely on the use of chemical pesticides and fertilizers, both of which have the potential to be harmful to the environment. Additionally, natural foods are typically sold in bulk, resulting in less wasteful packaging. Lastly, natural food consumption may also be a more moral choice. Fair trade practices are used to produce a lot of natural foods, which means that the people who grow and harvest these foods get paid a fair wage. This is significant on the grounds that it assists with supporting neighborhood networks and guarantees that laborers are dealt with decently. Moreover, normal food varieties are many times created utilizing others conscious cultivating strategies, and that implies that creatures are treated with deference and offered the chance to live in a common habitat.

All in all, there are many advantages to eating normal food varieties. These food sources are better, better for the climate, and can likewise be a more moral decision. Natural foods are definitely something you should think about if you want to improve your overall health and well-being or just help the environment. By doing the change to regular food varieties, you can partake in a better, more feasible eating routine that is great for yourself and really great for the planet.

CHAPTER3

What are the nutritional value of natural foods and processed foods

The nutritional value of and effects on human health of natural foods and processed foods are vastly different from one another. Foods that have undergone minimal processing and are devoid of additives, preservatives, and artificial flavors are considered natural foods. Handled food varieties, then again, are food varieties that have gone through critical handling and contain many added substances and additives. In this article, we will contrast normal food sources with handled food sources and make sense of why picking regular food sources for a solid diet is fundamental.

Natural foods are a great way to get the nutrients you need to be healthy. They are plentiful in nutrients, minerals, and other fundamental supplements that are important for ideal wellbeing. When compared to processed foods, the nutrients in natural foods are frequently more bioavailable, which means that they are easier for the body to absorb and utilize. Handled food varieties, then again, are many times high in calories, sodium, sugar, and unfortunate fats, which can prompt weight gain and other medical conditions. Notwithstanding their healthy benefit, normal food sources are likewise more harmless to the ecosystem than handled food varieties. Normal food varieties are many times developed utilizing feasible cultivating rehearses, which are better for the climate and help to protect regular assets. In contrast, industrial farming methods are frequently used to produce processed foods, which can be harmful to the environment due to the use of pesticides and other chemicals.

All in all, normal food varieties are a better and all the more harmless to the ecosystem choice contrasted with handled food varieties. They are easy to digest, full of vital nutrients, and good for your health as a whole. Natural foods are also a better choice for the environment and the environment, and they are more sustainable. Therefore, for a diet that is both healthy and long-lasting, natural foods must be preferred to processed foods.

The study of nourishment is a multidisciplinary field that incorporates the investigation of what food means for the human body, including the cycles of processing, ingestion, digestion, and end. Understanding the effects of nutrient deficiencies or excesses on the body and their role in overall health maintenance are also necessary. Nutrition science is a crucial part of clinical medicine, public health, sports performance, and other fields.

The study of sustenance is established in a huge collection of examination from various disciplines, including organic chemistry, physiology, microbial science, and brain research. This research has helped to identify the nutrients that are necessary for health and has improved our comprehension of the intricate interactions that take place between food and the human body. The development of interventions to encourage healthy eating habits and the investigation of dietary patterns and their effects on health outcomes are also part of nutrition science.

By and large, the study of nourishment is a quickly developing field that is basic for working on general wellbeing and forestalling persistent infections. As how we might interpret the perplexing connections among food and the human body keeps on developing, it will be fundamental to apply this information to foster successful procedures for advancing smart dieting propensities and diminishing the weight of diet-related illnesses. Through continuous examination and government funded schooling, sustenance science can possibly change the manner in which we ponder food and its effect on our healt

Nourishment is the investigation of what food means for the body and the connection between food, wellbeing, and sickness. A science manages supplements, the substances that food sources give to the body that are fundamental for development, upkeep, and fix. Natural foods have a lot of nutrients and can give the body everything it needs to work well. Natural foods contain protein, carbohydrates, vitamins, and minerals, which are the four main nutrients.

The body's muscles, organs, and bones all depend on protein for building and repairing tissues.

It is also needed to make enzymes, hormones, and other molecules that control how the body works. Protein can be tracked down in different regular food varieties, including meat, fish, eggs, dairy items, beans, and nuts. In order to ensure that the body receives all of the necessary amino acids, it is essential to consume a variety of protein sources.

The body's primary energy source is carbohydrates. They are essential for normal bodily functions and serve as fuel for the brain and muscles. Natural foods like fruits, vegetables, whole grains, and legumes contain carbohydrates. It is essential to pick complex sugars over straightforward carbs, as they give more supported

Energy and are less inclined to cause spikes in glucose levels.

Nutrients and minerals are fundamental for keeping up with great wellbeing and forestalling illness. They are necessary for the immune system, nervous system, and metabolism, among other bodily functions. Nutrients and minerals can be tracked down in various regular food sources, including natural products, vegetables, entire grains, and lean proteins. To ensure that the body receives all of the nutrients it requires, it is essential to consume a variety of these foods. Vitamin and mineral intake can aid in the prevention of chronic diseases like diabetes, cancer, and heart disease.

The study of how the body uses nutrients and how food affects health is called nutrition science. It is essential to comprehend the study of nourishment since it can assist us with settling on informed conclusions about what we eat and how we deal with our bodies. The significance of eating a well-balanced diet is one important aspect of nutrition. A diet that includes a variety of foods from all food groups in appropriate quantities is considered to be balanced.

A decent eating regimen is significant for some reasons. It supplies the nutrients the body requires to function properly. These supplements incorporate sugars, proteins, fats, nutrients, and minerals. A well-balanced diet will ensure that you get enough of each of these nutrients because they each play a specific role in the body. Carbohydrates, for instance, provide energy, while proteins are crucial for tissue building and repair. Vitamins and minerals are necessary for numerous bodily functions, while fats are essential for hormone production and brain function.

A decent eating routine can likewise assist with forestalling ongoing infections. Heart disease, stroke, diabetes, and some types of cancer can all be reduced by eating a diet high in fruits, vegetables, whole grains, and lean proteins. A fair eating regimen can likewise assist with keeping a sound weight, which is significant for in general wellbeing. By eating a fair eating routine and keeping a solid weight, you can lessen your gamble of creating numerous ongoing illnesses and carry on with a more drawn out, better life. In conclusion, a healthy diet that is well-balanced is important. It can aid in the prevention of long-term illnesses by providing the nutrients the body requires to function properly. You can ensure that your body gets the nutrients it needs to thrive by eating a variety of foods from all food groups and making healthy food choices.

Making a reasonable dinner plan is a fundamental part of keeping a sound way of life. A decent feast plan ought to incorporate supplements that come from starches, proteins, and fats. Proteins aid in the construction and repair of tissues, carbohydrates provide the body with the energy it needs to function, and fats aid in the absorption and storage of nutrients. Vitamins and minerals that are necessary for the body's growth and development should be included in a balanced diet.

To make a decent dinner plan, one ought to begin by figuring out the healthful necessities of their body. Meal plans will differ depending on each person's nutritional requirements.

The age, orientation, weight, and active work of an individual are a portion of the variables that decide their healthful requirements. Planning meals can begin once a person has identified their nutritional requirements. A variety of foods should be included in a balanced meal plan to ensure that all necessary nutrients are consumed.

To make a fair dinner plan, one ought to expect to incorporate various food sources from various nutritional categories. Fruits, vegetables, grains, proteins, and dairy are all part of the food groups. Since the body needs different nutrients from each food group, it's important to include foods from all food groups in a meal plan. A fair feast plan ought to likewise incorporate quality food decisions. These incorporate entire grains, lean proteins, low-fat dairy items, and solid fats. Quality food decisions give the body the fundamental supplements without adding abundance calories.

All in all, making a reasonable dinner plan is a significant part of keeping a sound way of life. Vitamins and minerals, in addition to carbohydrates, proteins, and fats, should be included in a well-balanced diet. Understanding one's nutritional requirements, aiming to include a variety of foods from various food groups, and selecting healthy food choices are all necessary steps in creating a balanced meal plan. By following a decent feast plan, people can guarantee that they are consuming the important supplements while keeping a sound weight.

Nourishment is the science that concentrates on the connection among food and the working of the body. It includes the body's metabolism, absorption, digestion, ingestion, and excretion of nutrients. The job of sustenance in keeping up with great wellbeing is basic as it gives the fundamental supplements expected to the body to accurately work. Maintaining good health in general necessitates eating a well-balanced diet that includes all of the necessary nutrients.

Sustenance assumes a vital part in keeping up with great wellbeing. For optimal function, the body requires a variety of nutrients, including vitamins, minerals, carbohydrates, protein, and fats. The body's growth, development, and maintenance are dependent on these nutrients.

The body functions properly and the immune system is strong enough to fight off infections and diseases when a diet that is well-balanced and contains all of the necessary nutrients.

An absence of legitimate sustenance can prompt different medical conditions. Hunger, which is the absence of fundamental supplements, can cause huge medical problems, including hindered development, debilitated resistant framework, and even demise. Then again, overconsumption of specific supplements can prompt weight, coronary illness, and other persistent ailments. Subsequently, it is fundamental to keep a decent eating routine that gives every one of the essential supplements in the perfect adds up to keep up with great wellbeing. In conclusion, the significance of nutrition in health maintenance cannot be overstated. A fair eating routine with every one of the expected supplements is fundamental for ideal working of the body. A healthy lifestyle necessitates a healthy diet and regular exercise, which can long-term prevent a variety of health issues.

Feast arranging is a fundamental part of solid living. It involves planning meals and snacks in advance to ensure that they are nutritious, delicious, and well-balanced. Natural food meal planning is a great way to ensure that your meals are nutritious and free of artificial ingredients. Foods that are grown or raised without the use of synthetic fertilizers, pesticides, or genetically modified organisms are known as natural foods.

Vitamins, minerals, and fiber are excellent sources of essential nutrients in natural foods. They are also low in fat and calories, making them ideal for people who want to lose weight or keep their current weight healthy. Choosing a variety of foods from various food groups, such as fruits, vegetables, whole grains, lean protein, and healthy fats, is an important part of meal planning with natural foods. Along these lines, you can make a fair feast that gives every one of the supplements your body needs.

CHAPTER 4

Planning meals with natural foods

Planning meals with natural foods is good for your health and the environment at the same time. By picking regular food sources, you are supporting manageable farming and diminishing the utilization of unsafe synthetic compounds in food creation. Additionally, natural foods are frequently less expensive than processed foods, making them an excellent choice for those on a tight budget. Generally, feast arranging with regular food sources is an extraordinary method for dealing with your wellbeing while likewise supporting the climate and setting aside cash.

With regards to dinner arranging, consolidating regular food varieties can carry a scope of advantages to your wellbeing, health, and generally speaking personal satisfaction. Regular food varieties are those that are insignificantly handled, liberated from fake fixings and added substances, and as near their normal state as could be expected. These food sources are frequently loaded with fundamental supplements, nutrients, and minerals that our bodies need to work at their best. There are a variety of advantages that can have a positive effect on our overall health and wellness if we place a high value on natural foods when planning our meals.

When planning meals, one of the primary advantages of natural foods is improved digestion and gut health. Fiber, which is essential for maintaining a healthy and functioning digestive system, is typically abundant in natural foods. Whole grains, legumes, fruits, and vegetables are all good sources of fiber, and planning your meals around them can help keep your gut happy and healthy. Moreover, normal food varieties are frequently simpler for our bodies to process, which can assist with lessening irritation, bulging, and other stomach related issues.

Natural foods also help with meal planning because they give you more energy and help you think clearly. Our bodies are able to access the nutrients they require to function at their best when we consume natural, whole foods. This can assist with further developing our energy levels, mental clearness, and in general concentration over the course of the day. By focusing on regular food sources in your dinner arranging, you might find that you have more energy, feel more ready, and are better ready to focus on your day to day assignments.

At last, integrating regular food varieties into your dinner arranging can assist with supporting a sound safe framework. Vitamins and minerals like zinc, vitamin D, and vitamin C, which are necessary for immune function, are frequently found in abundance in natural foods. At the point when we focus on these food sources in our dinner arranging, we can assist with supporting a sound safe framework that is better prepared to fend off diseases and contaminations. This can be particularly significant during cold and influenza season or seasons of high pressure or travel.

A healthy lifestyle necessitates meal planning with natural foods. You can make sure that you're getting all the nutrients your body needs to work properly when you plan your meals. Grocery shopping is an essential part of meal planning. To ensure that you have fresh, healthy, and nutrient-dense ingredients to prepare meals, it is essential to know how to shop for natural foods. Natural food grocery shopping tips are provided below.

In the first place, begin by making a rundown of the regular food varieties you want prior to going to the supermarket. Whole grains, fruits, vegetables, nuts, seeds, and lean meats ought to be on this list. You won't have to buy unhealthy food that isn't on your list this way. Likewise, you can save time by not meandering the store capriciously. It is vital for adhere to your rundown to guarantee that you are purchasing sound and normal food sources.

Second, pick privately developed and natural food varieties. Fresh local produce also helps local farmers. Pesticides, hormones, and other harmful chemicals are not present in organic foods. Organic produce is preferable because it contains more nutrients and is better for the body. You can find natural produce in a different part of the supermarket or at a neighborhood rancher's market.

Ultimately, read food names cautiously. Try to check the fixings rundown to guarantee that the food thing contains normal fixings. Avoid processed foods with artificial flavors, preservatives, and additives. Natural foods that are high in fiber, low in calories, and full of nutrients are your best bet. By following these shopping for food tips, you can guarantee that you are purchasing normal and good food sources for your dinner arranging.

Natural food meal planning is becoming increasingly popular as people seek healthier and more sustainable eating options. One significant part of feast arranging with normal food sources is dinner readiness. This entails selecting the appropriate ingredients and preparing them so that their inherent goodness and flavor are preserved. Natural meal preparation tips are provided below.

First and foremost, it is essential to select whole, fresh, and in season foods. This guarantees that your ingredients contain the most flavor and nutrients possible. A good rule of thumb is to keep things simple when preparing these ingredients. You should steer clear of thick sauces and a lot of butter or oils because both of these things can make your food more calorie- and fat-heavy.

One more key part of dinner planning with regular food varieties is cooking techniques. Natural foods can be cooked in a variety of ways to preserve their natural flavors and nutrients, including grilling, baking, and steaming. Abstain from profound searing or unreasonably heating up your fixings, as this can strip them of their supplements and make them less sound.

CHAPTER5

feast arrangement with Natural food varieties

Generally speaking, feast arrangement with normal food varieties is tied in with picking the right fixings, keeping things straightforward, and utilizing cooking techniques that save the regular decency of your food. You can savor delicious meals that are good for your body and the environment by doing this. Natural foods can play a significant role in achieving the goal of balanced meal planning, which is essential for maintaining a healthy diet and lifestyle. While arranging your feasts, it means a lot to zero in on consolidating various entire, supplement thick food varieties into your eating routine, including natural products, vegetables, entire grains, lean proteins, and sound fats. The vitamins, minerals, and nutrients your body needs to function properly and remain healthy are provided by these foods.

One method for guaranteeing that your feasts are adjusted is by utilizing the plate technique. Divide your plate into four sections using this method: one for lean protein, one for entire grains, and two for products of the soil. Healthy fats like avocado and olive oil can also be added to your plate in small amounts. In order to ensure that you get a variety of nutrients, aim for a variety of colors on your plate, which is another helpful tip. By observing these rules, you can make heavenly and nutritious dinners that will keep you feeling fulfilled and empowered over the course of the day.

With regards to regular food sources, there are numerous choices to look over. Because they contain a wide variety of vitamins, minerals, and antioxidants, fruits and vegetables are an excellent starting point. Entire grains, like earthy colored rice, quinoa, and entire wheat bread, are additionally significant for giving fiber and other fundamental supplements. Tofu, chicken, and other lean proteins like fish can support muscle growth and repair. Finally, brain function and overall health are dependent on healthy fats like avocados, nuts, and seeds. You can create a well-rounded and balanced diet that will support your health and well-being by incorporating these natural foods into your meal planning.

CHAPTER6

What are the natural food recipes

As people become more health-conscious and concerned about the quality of the ingredients in their food, natural food recipes are gaining popularity. Ingredients used in natural food recipes have been minimally processed and do not contain any artificial additives, preservatives, or chemicals. Whole foods, like fruits, vegetables, whole grains, nuts, and seeds, are the focus of these recipes, which aim to make meals that are both delicious and filling.

Natural food recipes offer a wide range of health benefits, which is one of the main advantages. Natural food recipes are loaded with vital vitamins, minerals, and nutrients that are necessary for optimal health because they use whole foods. These recipes likewise will quite often be lower in calories and fat, making them ideal for those hoping to keep a solid weight or get thinner. Natural food recipes are also frequently free of dairy, gluten, and other allergens, making them suitable for individuals with particular dietary restrictions.

One more advantage of regular food recipes is that they are unbelievably flexible and can be adjusted to suit many preferences and inclinations. Whether you lean toward exquisite or sweet, hot or gentle, there is a characteristic food recipe out there that will suit your necessities. Natural food recipes can also be made by grilling, roasting, baking, sautéing, and other methods, making them suitable for a wide range of cooking styles and methods.

All in all, normal food recipes are a fabulous method for working on your wellbeing and prosperity while as yet getting a charge out of heavenly and nutritious dinners. Natural food recipes provide a wide range of benefits that are certain to meet your needs, whether you are looking to maintain a healthy weight, improve your overall health, or simply enjoy delicious and healthy food. So, why not give them a shot right now and see for yourself all the amazing advantages of natural food recipes?

As more people try to eat healthier, natural food recipes have become increasingly popular. Natural food ingredients are free of harmful chemicals and additives that are typically found in processed foods, which is one of their main advantages. Not only are these chemicals harmful, but they also have the potential to cause allergies, obesity, and even cancer. By involving regular fixings in our food, we can be guaranteed of their virtue and partake in their healthy goodness.

Natural food ingredients' high nutrient content is yet another benefit. Dissimilar to handled food sources that are frequently deprived of their supplements during creation, normal fixings hold their regular nutrients, minerals, and cancer prevention agents. These nutrients are necessary for our overall health and well-being and can aid in the prevention of chronic diseases like diabetes, cancer, and heart disease. Natural ingredients can assist us in achieving optimal health and vitality if we include them in our diet.

At long last, normal food fixings are flexible and can be utilized in various recipes. When it comes to incorporating natural ingredients into our meals, there are endless options—from salads to soups, smoothies to desserts. In addition to adding flavor and texture, they offer a variety of health benefits that are not found in processed foods. By trying different things with various normal fixings, we can make tasty and nutritious dinners that are really great for our bodies, yet in addition fulfill our taste buds.

Natural food recipes are a great way to make healthy eating a part of your daily routine. Whole, unprocessed foods are used in these recipes, and there are no chemicals or additives in them.

You can prevent chronic diseases and improve your overall health and well-being by eating natural foods. Natural food recipes are one of the best because they are easy to make and can be altered to suit your preferences.

Natural food recipes that are easy to make are a great way to start eating healthy. These recipes utilize a couple of fixings and are not difficult to make, in any event, for the people who are not positive about the kitchen. Smoothie bowls, quinoa salads, and roasted vegetables are all examples of simple natural food recipes. These recipes are delectable as well as loaded with fundamental supplements that are useful for your body.

Simple natural food recipes have the advantage of being able to be prepared ahead of time and stored in the refrigerator for later use. This is especially helpful for people who are always on the go and don't have much time to cook during the week. You can guarantee that you will always have access to healthy and nutritious food if you prepare your meals in advance. Moreover, straightforward normal food recipes are in many cases spending plan well disposed, making them available to each and every individual who needs to eat better.

In conclusion, simple recipes using natural foods are a great way to boost your health and diet. Even for novice cooks, these recipes make use of whole, unprocessed ingredients and are simple to make. You can enjoy numerous health benefits and enhance your overall wellbeing by incorporating natural food recipes into your daily routine. So why not check these recipes out and see with your own eyes how tasty and nutritious they can be?

Natural food consumption is an essential component of a healthy lifestyle. Regular food varieties are those that come from nature and have not gone through any handling or alteration. They are full of vitamins, minerals, and nutrients that our bodies need to work at their best. Plant-based foods, such as fruits, vegetables, nuts, and seeds, can be incorporated into daily meals as one method of incorporating natural foods. In addition to being delicious, these foods have numerous health benefits.

CHAPTER7

Method for integrating regular food sources

One more method for integrating regular food sources into everyday dinners is by choosing entire grain items. The entire grain, including the bran, germ, and endosperm, is used to make whole grain products. They are high in fiber, which aids in maintaining a full and satisfied stomach. Instances of entire grain items incorporate earthy colored rice, quinoa, entire wheat bread, and oats. These items, which can be added to salads, soups, and stir-fries, are not only delicious but also nutritious.

Finally, integrating normal food varieties into day to day feasts can be made simple by involving them alternative for handled food sources. For instance, natural sweeteners like honey, maple syrup, and stevia can be utilized in place of processed sugar. Natural sweeteners are better for you and don't have the negative effects of processed sugar. In a similar vein, natural oils like olive oil, coconut oil, and avocado oil can be utilized in place of processed oils like canola oil. In addition to being healthier, these oils enhance the flavor of meals.

In conclusion, it is simple to ensure a healthy and balanced diet by incorporating natural foods into daily meals. One can reap the numerous health benefits of natural foods by incorporating plant-based foods, whole grain products, and natural alternatives to processed foods. It's important to remember that natural food consumption does not have to be difficult or costly. The preparation of natural foods can be a daunting task, particularly if you are not accustomed to cooking from scratch. Simple changes such as substituting natural foods for processed foods can go a long way toward promoting a healthy lifestyle. However, you can quickly learn how to use natural ingredients to make delicious and healthy meals with a few helpful hints. Investing in high-quality cookware that is long-lasting and simple to clean is one recommendation. Cooking will be easier and more enjoyable as a result of this. Learn how to wash, chop, and store fruits and vegetables correctly to preserve their nutrients and flavor is another helpful tidbit.

It is essential to experiment with various flavors and cooking techniques when preparing natural foods. Instead of relying on processed sauces and seasonings, one trick is to use fresh herbs and spices to enhance the flavor of your dishes. You can also try grilling or roasting your vegetables to make them sweeter and have a texture that is more satisfying. Using healthy fats like olive oil or avocado oil in place of vegetable oils or margarine, which can have a lot of trans fats and are bad for your health, is another trick.

Last but not least, it's important to make a grocery list and plan your meals ahead of time to make sure you have everything you need. This will help you avoid the temptation of unhealthy fast food and pre-packaged meals while also saving you time and money. To make healthy eating more convenient and sustainable, you can also try batch cooking and meal prepping. You can easily incorporate natural foods into your diet and reap all of their health benefits with these hints and tricks.

THE   END

www.ingramcontent.com/pod-product-compliance
Lightning Source LLC
Chambersburg PA
CBHW070040260726
48658CB00002B/675